Distribution, publication, and copying in any form are prohibited and subject to damages.

TEN HYPNOSES

Copying, publishing, and sharing with third parties are only permitted with the written consent of the author. Please observe the notes on copyright and usage.

Distribution, publication, and copying in any form are prohibited and subject to damages.

Copying, publishing, and sharing with third parties are only permitted with the written consent of the author. Please observe the notes on copyright and usage.

Distribution, publication, and copying in any form are prohibited and subject to damages.

Ingo Michael Simon

TEN HYPNOSES

6

SUICIDAL THOUGHTS AND ATTEMPTS

Copying, publishing, and sharing with third parties are only permitted with the written consent of the author. Please observe the notes on copyright and usage.

Distribution, publication, and copying in any form are prohibited and subject to damages.

© 2024 Ingo Michael Simon
All rights reserved.
Independently published
www.ingosimon.com

Important Notes for Urgent Attention:
The contents of this book are based on the practical experiences of the author with hypnosis applications and psychotherapy in a trance state. Although the author has strived for the utmost care, errors or misunderstandings in the presentation cannot be completely excluded. Therapeutic work with people and the application of hypnosis are solely the responsibility of the hypnotist. It cannot be ruled out that parts of this book may be misunderstood or that the application of a presented procedure may cause an undesirable reaction in the client. The author also assumes no co-responsibility if work with a client is carried out with reference to the statements in this book.

The Author:
Ingo Michael Simon studied psychology and education and is a hypnotherapist with practices in southwestern Germany and Switzerland. With the help of hypnosis-supported psychotherapy, he primarily treats people with persistent psychological conditions. His practice focuses on anxiety disorders, pathological compulsions, and psychosomatic illnesses. His therapeutic offerings mainly include classical and modern hypnosis applications and the dreamland therapy he developed himself.

Copying, publishing, and sharing with third parties are only permitted with the written consent of the author. Please observe the notes on copyright and usage.

Distribution, publication, and copying in any form are prohibited and subject to damages.

Notes on Copyright and Usage

Copying, publishing, and sharing with third parties is prohibited and only permitted with the written consent of the author. Please observe the following copyright and usage guidelines.

This work has been carefully crafted and created to the best of the author's knowledge and personal experience. It comprises text templates and application guidelines for professional hypnosis sessions. The author is a licensed psychotherapist with extensive experience in psychotherapy, coaching, and personal training using hypnotic techniques and methods. Nevertheless, the author and the publisher assume no liability for the accuracy of information, instructions, and advice, nor for any typographical errors. The author and publisher accept no responsibility or liability for the application of these texts and recommendations with clients or patients, nor for any potential consequences or unexpected reactions. It is expressly noted that the application of therapeutic and advisory techniques and formulations lies solely and entirely within the responsibility of the practitioner. This also applies to adherence to the boundaries of legally regulated medical and therapeutic practices. The fact that a book containing action proposals is freely available for sale does not imply that its application with clients or patients is permitted for everyone.

Copying, publishing, and sharing with third parties are only permitted with the written consent of the author. Please observe the notes on copyright and usage.

Distribution, publication, and copying in any form are prohibited and subject to damages.

Copying, publishing, and sharing with third parties are only permitted with the written consent of the author. Please observe the notes on copyright and usage.

Distribution, publication, and copying in any form are prohibited and subject to damages.

Table of contents

Introduction 9

#1 11

#2 15

#3 19

#4 24

#5 29

#6 34

#7 39

#8 45

#9 50

#10 55

Overview of All Titles in the Series "Ten Hypnoses" 60

Copying, publishing, and sharing with third parties are only permitted with the written consent of the author. Please observe the notes on copyright and usage.

Distribution, publication, and copying in any form are prohibited and subject to damages.

Copying, publishing, and sharing with third parties are only permitted with the written consent of the author. Please observe the notes on copyright and usage.

Introduction

The series "Ten Hypnoses" is very well known in Germany, Austria, and Switzerland as a collection of texts for therapeutic work and is used by numerous psychotherapeutic practices, doctors, therapists, coaches, and other helping professionals. I am pleased to now be able to offer these texts in other countries as well.

Most therapists have their own methods for inducing and deepening trance as well as for exiting trance. Therefore, I have focused on the main part of the hypnosis. The texts in this book can be integrated as the main part into any hypnosis process.

The texts in this collection use various hypnosis techniques. I will not explain these in detail, as I assume that users have the appropriate training. It is also not necessary to understand the exact structure or functioning of the different parts. The texts can simply be read aloud, and they will have their effect.

Decide for yourself which text best suits your client or patient at any given time. You can also combine passages from different texts. It is not about using all ten hypnoses in sequence. It is a selection of possibilities.

I want to emphasize that books cannot replace therapy. Psychotherapy or other therapeutic treatments involve much more. A careful diagnosis is the necessary basis for deciding on the use of methods, including whether hypnosis or one of my texts should be used. Even in this case, preparatory discussions, follow-up discussions during the session, and of course, a therapeutic concept for the sequence of sessions and the content approaches are essential parts of therapy. This cannot and should not be achieved with a collection of texts.

In any case, I wish you much success in your work and I am pleased if my text templates can contribute in a small way.

Ingo Michael Simon

#1

For Affected Individuals

You survived... Your despair had brought you to the point of wanting to end your life, but you survived... Now, you are rediscovering the meaning of your life... finding new goals... new paths... new courage to live... It's truly remarkable how well you are now able to focus on life again...

...... Let's begin with life in the here and now... with life in this very moment... Feel inside yourself and notice how relaxed you can be at this moment... so calm and composed, in this beautiful trance... in this state of relaxation and peace... Only this feeling matters now... Let it become very clear... focus more intensely on it and you will realize that this is exactly the peace you have been seeking... The clearer you can feel the inner peace you now experience, the more conscious you become that this is the peace you were searching for... It's truly remarkable that you can find and feel this deep peace within yourself so clearly... Some time ago, you sought peace and thought you could no longer find it in this life... But you can... right now, everything within you is calm... You can now rest... give yourself time and regain new strength... It's wonderful that you have managed to find the peace you need... It's good that you have found this inner peace at this moment... So it is possible to find peace in life... It is possible to find distance from everyday life in life... It is also possible to find balance and relaxation in life... just like now... exactly like now... You can do it... You have already done it...

... ... And if it is possible now, it will be possible again and again... Every day, you can find this peace within yourself by doing exactly what you did today... In complete calm... at your own pace... in your own time, you can enter the state of inner peace and tranquility... just like now...

... ... Now, you can focus on yourself and find new goals... You feel that your new life goal is waiting deep within you... It waits for you in the peace and tells you: You survived, discover life anew... Perhaps that is the special goal within you... Discover life anew... your life... your own life...

... ... With each breath, you can come closer to your will to live... With each breath, you take in strength and joy of living... the will to continue living and to discover life anew...

Each time you inhale, you gain more strength... feel your inner strength becoming stronger... Feel every breath consciously, and then you can feel it precisely... Each inhale brings you strength and courage... The more you focus on inhaling, the more clearly you can feel that you actually find strength and new courage... So, breathe consciously and deliberately now... Breathe deeply and feel the strength... Breathe deeply and feel the courage... Breathe deeply and feel the will to survive... Breathe deeply and feel your own strength growing... becoming larger and more stable with each breath... larger and more stable... with each breath, feel the strength...

... ... [Speak the following suggestive words in sync with the client's breathing, always during the inhalation] ... ...

... ... Strength... Courage... Will to live... ... ... Strength... Courage... Will to live... ... ... Strength... Courage... Will to live... ... ... Strength... Courage... Will to live... ... ... Strength... Courage... Will to live...

... ... Good... That's right... You're doing it right... Now rest and stay in your strength for a minute until you hear my voice again...

... ... [Pause for about a minute, let the client breathe calmly, then continue reading, not paying attention to the breathing rhythm] ... ...

Now, you have already gained a lot... You survived and that is your goal for the coming time... survive... continue living... shape your life again... Today, you focus on this as best you can with all your newly gained strength... This new strength makes it especially easy for you to value and cherish yourself... to always accept and love yourself... to be there for yourself...

All these words are deeply anchored in your subconscious... Everything imprints itself deeply in your feelings... So every day, if you want, you can breathe consciously for your life and breathe for your inner courage... Whenever you breathe slowly and deeply because you want to live, you immediately feel the inner strength... the growing strength... You simply breathe slowly and deeply and feel your life force...

Whenever you feel that you need more strength and courage for your life, you just breathe slowly and deeply...

slowly and deeply... and feel your strength and your courage... just like today... exactly like today...

#2

For Affected Individuals

You have realized that your own life must go on... You have lost a loved one who ended their life, and you have asked yourself a thousand times if it could have been different... why this person could not continue living... But now, you are also taking care of yourself because your life goes on... and you have a right to a happy and free life... today and every day of your life... Your life goes on... It is important to let go now... everything that can hold you back in your life... so that you can move forward again... into your life because your life goes on...

... ... Focus on your breathing and imagine that you can let go of every burden with your breath... You know this from your everyday life, like everyone does... When we are burdened and want to free ourselves, we breathe in deeply and exhale strongly and for a long time... Then we feel freer and find new strength and new courage... That is exactly what you need most now... strength and courage... So breathe consciously and deliberately... and let go of everything that could hold you back... everything that burdens you... everything that could prevent you from feeling free...

...... First, let go of the guilt, because you could not prevent it... Breathe in deeply and exhale strongly and let go of the guilt...

...... [Let the client breathe in and out calmly once, then repeat the process together] ......

...... once more... ...

...... [Breathe in deeply with the client and speak the next word with a clear exhale; "breathe" the word out clearly!] ......

...... Let go!... ...

...... Now let go of the feeling of guilt, because you are not responsible... Breathe in deeply and exhale strongly and let go of the feeling of guilt...

...... [Let the client breathe in and out calmly once, then repeat the process together] ......

...... once more... ...

... ... [Breathe in deeply with the client and speak the next word with a clear exhale; "breathe" the word out clearly!] ... ...

... ... Let go!... ...

... ... Now let go of the anger and rage, because deep down, you are sad... Breathe in deeply and exhale strongly and let go of the anger and rage...

... ... [Let the client breathe in and out calmly once, then repeat the process together] ... ...

... ... once more... ...

... ... [Breathe in deeply with the client and speak the next word with a clear exhale; "breathe" the word out clearly!] ... ...

... ... Let go!... ...

... ... Now let go of the sadness, because you are allowed to be happy again... Breathe in deeply and exhale strongly and let go of the sadness...

... ... [Let the client breathe in and out calmly once, then repeat the process together] ... ...

… … once more… …

… … [Breathe in deeply with the client and speak the next word with a clear exhale; "breathe" the word out clearly!] … …

… … Let go!… …

All these words are deeply anchored in your subconscious… Everything imprints itself deeply in your feelings… So every day, if you want, you can breathe consciously for your letting go and breathe for your inner freedom… Whenever you breathe out slowly and deeply because you want to let go, you immediately feel the inner liberation… the lightness… You simply breathe slowly and deeply and feel your letting go…

Whenever you feel that old thoughts could come back, you just breathe slowly and deeply… slowly and deeply… and let go… just like today… exactly like today…

#3

For Affected Individuals

The following hypnosis session works with an olfactory anchor (scent anchor). An anchor is a trigger that should evoke a specific feeling or thought. We want to help the client strengthen their courage to live with the help of a specific scent. We discuss this with the client before the session and keep a bottle with a scent ready. This can be a smelling oil or an aroma spray that the client should only smell in trance. During the hypnosis session, we then set the anchor by presenting the scent and associating it suggestively. The scent itself should not be too strong, but it does not have to be particularly pleasant for the client. It is about the suggestive connection. However, it should not be perceived as repulsive either. With mild aroma oils, this should hardly be the case. Main Part 4 uses the same hypnosis, adapted for work with relatives. As you will see, this can be done quite easily with "small" changes!

Living is your goal... You have firmly resolved to embrace life again and to find the strength within you to actively and confidently shape your life... to overcome your grief and despair again and again and to continue living... to find meaning in your life again... to discover goals worth living for... to find your goals and your contentment... You have succeeded in this again and again... because you are still alive, even though you have often thought about ending your life... This thought may come back, and then the question arises again... How can one best manage to live...

... ... Today we are working with an anchor, as we have discussed... Maybe you are already wondering how quickly this anchor will work... how quickly the scent you will soon get to know can immediately give you a sense of hope and confidence... It might surprise you how well this anchor works... how quickly you can actually come to a pleasant feeling of life, especially when it gets tough...

... ... Today is the first day of your new life... in a life where you can quickly reach a good feeling of life again and again... The good thing is that it is much easier than you thought before... Maybe you are wondering how best and quickest to feel a good feeling of life immediately... to feel courage to live and the will to live...

... ... It is easier than you thought... To do this, you now mentally go to a time when you felt really good, maybe the best time of your life... maybe it was a long span of time, several years... or there was a short period that was really nice... a vacation, an experience... maybe just a very short moment that was really nice... the best moment of your life... if you want, also take simply the best fantasy of your life... and go entirely into the feeling associated with it... feel once again how beautiful it was... The more you focus on your memory or your fantasy, the more intensely you can feel the good feeling of life... maybe freedom... lightness... joy... happiness... You feel really good in this memory... or in this fantasy... You feel better and better... The more you focus on your memory or your fantasy, the more intensely you can feel the good feeling of life... exactly like that... Let the feeling in you become more beautiful... Exactly this feeling you need... Exactly this feeling you need every day...

... ... You can secure it... You can ensure that you can do this in your waking everyday life too... just like now... every day just like now... It is very simple... You can go into this feeling every day and feel good... It succeeds again and again, especially when it gets tough... Then it suddenly becomes easy to feel the good feeling of life... Then it suddenly becomes easy to choose life...

...... [Open the bottle with the aroma and move it towards the client's nose; hold it there] ......

Now take a deep breath and consciously perceive the scent you are sensing... a pleasant scent... at the same time, you feel very clearly that you actually want to live... Your good feeling and this scent you perceive now combine with each other... They belong together... This scent and wanting to live belong very closely together... This scent means: Yes, I want to live! ... Yes, I want to live! ... Take another deep breath... The scent of life spreads through you... The scent of life flows through your entire body... from your nose to your lungs... into your upper body... into your abdomen and into your legs... Life flows through you completely... Life flows through you completely...

...... And whenever you smell this scent, you feel alive... Whenever you perceive this very scent, you feel very clearly that you want to live... Even when you only think of the scent, you can already feel that you want to live... Your subconscious imprints this scent and associates it with the best time of your life... with life... with life...

... ... [Now remove and close the bottle] ... ...

... ... Continue to breathe calmly and enjoy the peace... Give yourself now mindfulness and attention and trust your subconscious, which helps you to get into this state very quickly by simply smelling the bottle with the scent I just presented to you...

You can even test it... As soon as you perceive the scent, you feel good and want to live... It's like breathing life in when you smell it... Inhaling this scent means breathing in life...

... ... [Open the bottle again and hold it to the client's nose so they can clearly perceive the scent; hold it briefly and then close it again] ... ...

... ... That feels good... very, very good... Your inner self imprints firmly that already reaching for the bottle with your personal scent of life triggers the signal in your body: Yes, I want to live! ... Yes, I want to live! ...

Distribution, publication, and copying in any form are prohibited and subject to damages.

Copying, publishing, and sharing with third parties are only permitted with the written consent of the author. Please observe the notes on copyright and usage.

#4

For Relatives

The following hypnosis session works with an olfactory anchor (scent anchor). An anchor is a trigger that should evoke a specific feeling or thought. We want to help the client strengthen their courage to live with the help of a specific scent. We discuss this with the client before the session and keep a bottle with a scent ready. This can be a smelling oil or an aroma spray that the client should only smell in trance. During the hypnosis session, we then set the anchor by presenting the scent and associating it suggestively. The scent itself should not be too strong, but it does not have to be particularly pleasant for the client. It is about the suggestive connection. However, it should not be perceived as repulsive either. With mild aroma oils, this should hardly be the case. Main Part 3 uses the same hypnosis, adapted for work with affected individuals. As you will see, this can be done quite easily with "small" changes!

Finding peace is your goal... You have firmly resolved to live your life constructively and to find the strength within you to actively and confidently shape your life... to overcome your grief and guilt again and again and to continue living... to find meaning in your life again... to discover things worth living for... to continue your path... You have succeeded in this again and again... because you have lost a person, but you are still alive, even if guilt feelings plague you... You are not responsible... You are allowed to grieve and cry, you are allowed to feel and express your feelings... You are allowed to free yourself from all self-reproach and guilt... You are allowed to find your inner peace again now...

... ... Today we are working with an anchor, as we have discussed... Maybe you are already wondering how quickly this anchor will work... how quickly the scent you will soon get to know can immediately give you a sense of inner peace and confidence... It might surprise you how well this anchor works... how quickly you can actually come to a pleasant feeling of life, especially when it gets tough...

... ... Today is the first day of your new life... in a life where you can quickly reach the feeling of inner peace again and again... The good thing is that it is much easier than you thought before... Maybe you are wondering how best and quickest to feel inner peace and confidence immediately... to feel courage to live and the will to live... It is easier than you thought... To do this, you now mentally go to a time when you felt really good, maybe the best time of your life... maybe it was a long span of time, several years... or there was a short period that was really nice... a vacation, an experience... maybe just a very short moment that was really nice... the best moment of your life... if you want, also take simply the best fantasy of your life... and go entirely into the feeling associated with it... feel once again how beautiful it was... The more you focus on your memory or your fantasy, the more intensely you can feel the good feeling of life... maybe freedom... lightness... joy... happiness... and your inner peace... You feel really good in this memory... or in this fantasy... You feel better and better... The more you focus on your memory or your fantasy, the more intensely you can feel the good feeling of inner peace... exactly like that... Let the feeling in you become more beautiful... Exactly this feeling you need... Exactly this feeling you need every day...

...... You can secure it... You can ensure that you can do this in your waking everyday life too... just like now... every day just like now... It is very simple... You can go into this feeling every day and feel good... It succeeds again and again, especially when it gets tough... Then it suddenly becomes easy to feel the good feeling of inner peace... Then it suddenly becomes easy to choose life...

... ... [Open the bottle with the aroma and move it towards the client's nose; hold it there] ... ...

Now take a deep breath and consciously perceive the scent you are sensing... a pleasant scent... at the same time, you feel very clearly that you actually want to live... Your good feeling of inner peace and this scent you perceive now combine with each other... They belong together... This scent and inner peace belong very closely together... This scent means: Yes, I find my peace! ... Yes, I find my peace! ... Take another deep breath... The scent of peace spreads through you... The scent of peace flows through your entire body... from your nose to your lungs... into your upper body... into your abdomen and into your legs... Peace flows through you completely... Peace flows through you completely... And whenever you smell this scent, you feel alive... Whenever you perceive this very scent, you feel very clearly your inner peace... Even when you only think of the scent, you can already feel that you become calmer... Your subconscious imprints this scent and associates it with the best time of your life... with peace... with inner peace...

... ... [Now remove and close the bottle] ... ...

... ... Continue to breathe calmly and enjoy the peace... Give yourself now mindfulness and attention and trust your subconscious, which helps you to get into this state very quickly by simply smelling the bottle with the scent I just presented to you...

You can even test it... As soon as you perceive the scent, you feel calmer and experience this peaceful feeling... It's like breathing in peace when you smell it... Inhaling this scent means breathing in peace...

... ... [Open the bottle again and hold it to the client's nose so they can clearly perceive the scent; hold it briefly and then close it again] ... ...

... ... That feels good... very, very good... Your inner self imprints firmly that already reaching for the bottle with your personal scent of peace triggers the signal in your body: Yes, I find my peace! ... Yes, I find my peace! ...

#5

For Affected Individuals

You know the thoughts about ending your life... Many times you have thought about ending your life... Maybe you are still unsure whether you want to continue living or choose another path... Basically, we all have to decide to live again and again... to keep going even when everything seems hopeless... In fact, we decide every day anew for life...

... ... Maybe you have encountered many people who claimed never to have thought about ending their life or wished to be dead and find peace... You may have then thought you were one of the few who really ever thought about it... or one of the few who already tried to end their life... But the truth is different... different, even though it is rarely spoken about this way... In truth, it is not about whether a person wants to continue living or die, but about how strong the respective desire is... Because every person thinks about it at some point and repeatedly, whether it would be better to find complete peace... That is completely normal… It is human… Most of the time, we then decide to continue living… You also made this decision because that's why you are here and want to understand everything better… want to find a way that brings you fully back to life… Maybe you also want to check whether it is really worth living…

… … Now you are in a state of relaxation and can think about everything in peace… very calmly and just for yourself find what makes your life worthwhile… what made it worthwhile before and what will make it worthwhile today and in the future… For this, imagine that you are in a cinema and make yourself really comfortable in the soft seat you are sitting in there… It is quite dark, but you can still see everything well… You are completely alone in this cinema so that you really have enough space for yourself, without being distracted or disturbed by anyone… Time and peace just for you…

… … The cinema screen is covered by a heavy curtain… which slowly opens… The curtain slowly slides to the side… and in a few moments, the movie of your life begins… like a movie trailer showing the best scenes of a film… you can view your own life… the already past part… but also what may come... The curtain slides to the side, and it becomes very quiet in your inner cinema... very quiet deep within you... This makes your movie a glimpse into your deepest self...

...... The movie begins... First, you see a bright square on the screen, just like before, and numbers run backwards, just like films were announced a long time ago... ten... nine... eight... seven... six... five... four... three... two... one... Your movie begins...

...... First, you see scenes from your childhood... You see yourself as a child... Let the images simply be there... maybe they are burdensome or painful... but they help you understand everything better... Just let the images be there, the ones that show up by themselves... Look at them, wherever you are now... It is a look into the past that is already over... Then you also see beautiful pictures from your childhood... maybe a favorite toy... a place where you felt safe... a person who was good to you... who protected and comforted you... You remember your plans and wishes... the dreams of your childhood... You feel the good feeling of the beautiful moments again… the good feeling of being safe, even if only for short moments… You feel this good feeling…

… … Then the scene jumps to your adult time… You see images that show how it came about that you wanted to end your life… Like in fast forward, you see again how everything developed and became more and more hopeless… how you made the decision to end your life… Now you are here in relaxation and peace… Now you can calmly view everything… maybe understand again how it was… Maybe you are happy now that you survived… that you did not end your life… And again the images of your life change… You see images that show you what is worth living for even today… You see images of the plans and ideas you have deep inside… of what you still want to do or experience… maybe things that are easy to reach, maybe also those that are a bit utopian… But once it was so that precisely the big fantasies could bring you to always dream with joy and imagine: What if you had the free choice… So you begin again now to dream and develop ideas of what you still want to experience… where you would like to go once… whom you would like to meet if you had the free choice... And with all these small or big dreams, you find many reachable goals that show you that there are still many worthwhile things and goals for you... At the same time, your will to live becomes stronger... You feel deep inside, if you pay close attention to your body feeling, this pleasant tension that shows you that you can still achieve so much... can be happy and stay happy... can live your life contentedly... Let all wishes and dreams become very clear and enjoy the bath in your own fantasy and creativity...

... ... And while you watch your inner pictures, you realize that fantasy and reality are very close together... sometimes even they are the same... So on any day, a truth can become of a beautiful fantasy... when you let your fantasy wander in your own dream pictures and imagine that you really have the free choice...

#6

For Relatives

You have lost someone who took their own life... ... You couldn't prevent it... ... It was his/her decision, but you have blamed yourself a thousand times for not noticing or you often thought you should have done something differently... ... to avert it... ... maybe you also thought it was your fault... ... Then there might have been anger and fury about what happened... ... So many emotions often get mixed up... ... and also the realization that what happened cannot be changed... ...

... ... Behind all the feelings of despair, anger, guilt, and reproach towards others, there is a particular feeling... ... the feeling of loss... ... the feeling of infinite sorrow... ... Today, it is only about this feeling because it is a very important one... ... So, today, let your grief be fully present... ... All other feelings become small when you can fully feel your sadness... ... It is what leads to all the reproaches and self-reproaches... ...

... ... You have already thought and imagined so much... ... always wondering: What if? ... ... But that was the holding on that made overcoming grief so difficult... ... You can learn from memories... ... and you have already learned everything there was to learn... ... Now you can let the memory be and let go at the same time... ... Now it is time to say goodbye to the what-if and focus on what is truly important... ... looking ahead... ... shaping your life here and now and every day... ...

Deep within you, there is the Place of Clarity... ... At this place, there is only white, pure light... ... You stand at this place and see light everywhere around you... ... Let this image become very clear... ... white light around you... ... only light everywhere... ... Immerse yourself completely in the vision of pure white light and complete inner freedom... ...

... ... The more intensely you imagine the white light, the easier it becomes to feel the inner freedom at this very moment... ... Now, in relaxation and calm, it is quite easy to feel the sense of inner freedom... ... because now everything feels calm... ... all problems are far away because now it is only about your peace... ... Now is the time just for you... ...

time just for you... ... Everywhere around you is white, pure light... ... Let it become clearer and clearer in your imagination... ... before your inner eye... ... white light and peace... ... white light and relaxation... ... white light and freedom... ... freedom... ...

... ... The ground beneath your feet seems glassy... ... you can see through it... ... infinitely deep... ... But even there you see only pleasant, white light... ... white light deep into infinity... ... You look up and see only light above you too... ... It is everywhere... ... bright and clear and very pleasant... ... It envelops you and gives you clarity and openness... ...

... ... You see a glass wall in front of you... ... You can look through it and see only light behind the wall... ... It is beautiful at the Place of Clarity... ... so pure... ... so free... ... so bright and clear... ... so distinct... ... You look at the wall in front of you again... ... In the light behind the wall, a shadow slowly appears... ... It is the shadow of a person coming closer and becoming more recognizable... ... Then you recognize the face and see this person you have lost, who ended their life because they couldn't act otherwise... ... Here at the Place of Clarity, you can meet this person... ...

... ... He/She looks completely unharmed, pure and clear, like in the best time of life... ... He/She radiates incredible peace... ... You stand very close to the wall... ... You can see him/her... ... He/She speaks to you... ... You can hear his/her voice... ... He/She thanks you because you have thought so much about him/her with your inner struggle... ... always wondering why he/she had to die and why you couldn't prevent it... ... He/She thanks you for this concern and tells you at the same time that you have thought and mourned enough for him/her... ... He/She tells you that he/she made this decision himself/herself and wants to take responsibility for it... ... Then you clearly hear the words... ... You are innocent... ... Live your life now... ... You are innocent... ... Live your life now... ...

Let these words flow into you... ... Let them take effect and give yourself peace and mindfulness... peace and mindfulness... ... You are innocent... ... Live your life now... ... Embrace yourself inwardly and feel the effect of the words you hear at the glass wall... ... You are innocent... ... Live your life now... ...

... ... Now say goodbye to the dear person on the other side of the glass wall... ... in complete peace... ...

This Place of Clarity is deep within you, and you can go there every day, whenever you want... ... Deep within you, you then hear the words... ... You are innocent... ... Live your life now... ... So you remember every day that you can continue to live in peace... ... again and again... ... and it is really simple... ... a glance in the mirror is enough... ... Every morning, when you look in the mirror, it is as if you are standing in front of the glass wall at the Place of Clarity and hear these words... ... You are innocent... ... Live your life now... ... You are innocent... ... Live your life now...

#7

For Relatives

Ideomotor response refers to the phenomenon that our body follows our feelings and thoughts with movements. In everyday life, this following manifests as body posture, muscle tension, and movement patterns of a person, which naturally change with the mood and thoughts. In trance, ideomotor signals can be used to obtain information that the client cannot actively communicate. The subconscious can answer questions with an agreed finger signal, for example. Of course, ideomotor responses can also be used suggestively, such as in arm levitation and catalepsy. Such an approach, which I also use in the following text, strengthens trust in hypnosis and one's ability to change, thereby promoting therapy.

You have lost a loved one who ended their own life... ... It was a shock for you, and you have often thought about how it could have come to this... ... Then you repeatedly blamed yourself, chastised yourself for not noticing it earlier... ... or you believed that you could or even should have prevented it... ... But you also know that every person decides for themselves... ... that you cannot stop someone who does not want to allow it... ... And as hard as it may sound... ... Everyone is responsible for their own actions... ... You did not kill him/her... ... You did not wish him/her dead... ... Whatever may have been... ... how much may have gone wrong... ... or passed by unnoticed by you all... ... It was not your fault that it happened this way... ... Some things are unavoidable, even if we often believe we could or should have avoided them... ... It was not your fault... ... Therefore, it is also time to let go of your guilt feelings today... ... perhaps as much as possible today and then repeatedly... ... It was not your fault, so I want to help you let go of your guilt feelings... ...

... ... You have understood that the guilt you felt was not truly yours, but you only believed you were guilty... Now you know better... You know that you are innocent... You therefore want to let go of the guilt feelings... In your thoughts, you have already succeeded, and that is really good... Now you can work on letting go of your guilt feelings...

Your deep inner self will do this for you... Your subconscious can plan anew for you and thereby ensure that you handle yourself more mindfully from the start and only take on the responsibility that truly belongs to you... To do this, you must allow your subconscious to help you... and that is exactly what you have already done by focusing on your inner peace and your body... So you have already sent your subconscious the message that it may now work quietly for you... a nice idea that it is not you who works, but your unconscious side... completely in silence... You allow it, and that is why it is also possible... Now focus your attention on your hands... Check once again that they are lying correctly next to your body... loose and comfortable... in complete relaxation... Your palms lightly touch the surface...

... [If the position has not been taken or has changed in the meantime, please correct it until the hands are lying loosely next to the body.] ...

Now your subconscious takes the lead... Your deep inner self ensures that old thought and behavior patterns that produced your bad conscience and guilt feelings fall away from you and that new thoughts of freedom are built up... completely without effort... in peace and quiet... Your subconscious ensures that you handle yourself and your inner resources more mindfully and lets this new mindfulness and self-care become a matter of course... It is like an inner cleansing... Old patterns of thinking and behavior are let go... new patterns of thinking and behavior are built up and help you to live more freely and happily from now on... to let go of guilt feelings promptly and sustainably... to work with peace and overview... to shape the day more calmly with trust in inner guidance...

... Your subconscious now shows you how quickly it progresses in this cleansing and renewal... You will recognize it by the fact that your hands will soon begin to turn outwards... Your hands slowly turn outwards until they finally lie on their backs... Focus on your hands and just let it happen... Your subconscious now begins to turn your hands outwards... slowly, at your pace, in your tempo... The more you adjust internally to your new thinking and acting, the more your hands turn... The more you let go of your bad conscience now, the more your hands turn... They turn more and more outwards... Your hands turn with every step of internal change and realignment... just like that... Feel how your hands slowly turn... They turn outwards... as if by themselves... You don't have to do anything... You don't have to undertake anything... You don't have to actively change anything... Your subconscious does everything necessary for you... And as a sign of letting go, your hands turn... more and more... further and further... until they show with the palms upwards...

... [Observe the turning of the hands, which starts relatively quickly. The client connects the turning with inner change. Repeat suggestions for turning the hands until they lie on their backs.] ...

Isn't it amazing how quickly your subconscious is ready to help you and even show you... Your inner self says to you: Yes, I am realigning internally... Yes, I am letting go of the old guilt feelings now... Yes, I am giving myself mindfulness and care... Yes, I am taking good care of myself from now on... Yes, I am innocent... Yes, I am innocent...

... ... Your inner self firmly imprints that you are now free and can take new paths... ... and whenever you want to strengthen the feeling of inner freedom, you can simply lay your hands next to your body and consciously turn them... ... You breathe out deeply and then feel the inner liberation, the letting go of all guilt feelings... ... You can do this every day of your life, if you want... ... whenever you want... ... and wherever you want... ... It is very simple...

#8

For Affected Individuals

Today you want to focus on your will to live, to find it and make it stronger again... ... Many times you almost lost it and thought about ending your life... ... Then you considered being able to live on if it was still worth living... ... So you are always searching for the meaning of continuing to live... ... for the courage to live on... ... and for the strength to continue living... ... That is what you need most... ... Vitality... ... Sometimes we feel this strength very clearly and deeply within us... ... Then we feel the will to live our life actively and with joy... ... Sometimes, too, we cannot really feel the deep strength within us that tells us: Accept the challenge of your life and persevere... ... So it can often go back and forth... ... But today it is about finding the deep strength of life within you, feeling how strong it really is... ... and recognizing that it is there even when you can hardly feel it... ... The strength lies in your soul, but it also shows in your body... ... as a feeling... ... as a physical sensation deep within you...

Every thought, every mood... ... every single feeling manifests in our body... ... shows itself there as warmth or coolness... ... as pressure or relaxation... ... as a strange feeling or as tingling... ... sometimes even as pain... ... So if you can feel your body clearly, you can achieve everything you have set out to do... ... find and clearly feel the strength of life... ... and change everything... ... let go of everything you want to leave in the past to be free and open again... ... find strength to accept life and look ahead... ... trust yourself and your abilities again... ... That will succeed today... ... and it will succeed every day of your life... ... every day...

... ... Somewhere in your body sits the strength of life... ... There also sits the courage that helps you get through difficult times again... ... There also sits the hope that carries you further... ... There also sits the confidence that you can make it and live... ... All this sits deep within you and has helped you survive without you noticing it... ... Because this strength... ... these many strengths within you led to you not doing it after all... ... that you decided again and again to live a little longer... ... All these helpful forces are anchored in your feelings and thoughts, but also in your body... ... You can feel them in your body... ... Maybe you know that you can feel everything that belongs to you physically when you come to rest, like now... ... and focus on your body... ... like now...

... ... Now direct your attention to your body and feel your body... ... Go from head to toe downwards, as if you were standing next to yourself and could look at your body... ... and find this special spot... ... Find this spot that feels somehow different because your strength lies there...

... ... In your imagination, you stand next to yourself and look at your body to find this special spot now... ... It is marked with a thick red dot... ... You see it before your inner eye... ... Just look at your body... ... Wherever this dot may be, it is exactly the spot on your body where your strength can best show itself, even if this spot doesn't feel particularly strong... ... Strength is often overlaid by our doubts... ... But it is there... ... exactly where you see the red dot before your inner eye or where you can best imagine it, because that is enough... ... You find the spot now... ... It is marked in red and feels different... ... maybe just a bit cooler or warmer... ... maybe as tingling... ... or as slight goosebumps that suddenly form... ... Wherever this spot is... ... There your vitality shows itself through a physical signal... ...

exactly there... ... But even if you haven't found it yet... ... It is there... ... Then just take the spot that spontaneously comes to mind... ... wherever that is... ... Feel deeper and deeper into it... ... It is your vitality waiting for you there in hiding...

... ... Now focus all your attention and all your mindfulness and loving care on exactly this spot of your body and connect with the inner pattern that lies there... ... Imagine how from this spot a warm feeling flows in all directions... ... as if an inner sun is at exactly this spot, spreading its light and warmth gently in all directions... ... Let it become warmer and warmer, as pleasant as possible... ... Imagine bright light radiating from this spot into the depths of your body... ... and also outwards... ... Let this spot of your body become a source of warmth and have an increasingly pleasant effect on you... ... This warmth can encompass your entire body because you bring this mindfulness... ... this turning towards yourself... ... So this spot of your body becomes ever calmer... ... ever more relaxed... ... ever more pleasant... ... and your vitality becomes stronger... ... More and more old entanglements are released and replaced by new patterns of self-care and mindfulness... ... You find more and more love from yourself for yourself... ... Self-love and mindfulness... ... Your vitality becomes stronger... ... Feel deeply into yourself... ... You find more and more love from yourself for yourself... ... Self-love and mindfulness... ... Your vitality becomes stronger... ... with each moment and with the concentration on your body... ... You find more and more love from yourself for yourself... ... Self-love and mindfulness... ... Your vitality becomes stronger

... ... Whenever you focus on your body and find a spot that feels distinctly different from the rest of your body, you give yourself mindfulness and focus on this spot... ... This way, you can strengthen your vitality, your courage, your hope, and also your confidence... ... This way, you can live...

#9

For Affected Individuals

You go into the land of dreams... ... You stand on a wide path, and your legs begin to walk as if by themselves... ... You follow this path through the land of your dreams, not knowing where it can lead you... ... It is completely quiet because no one but you is on this path... ... So you have the freedom to walk at your own pace... ... to follow only yourself... ... You don't have to wait for anyone or follow anyone... ... So this path can become a very personal path... ... especially a path to yourself...

... ... You look around and see nature wherever you look... ... Everything looks untouched and new, as if this land of dreams has just been created... ... And maybe that is exactly how it is. Maybe this land is just being created with every step... ... And with each step further on your path, you discover something new that is just being created... ... deep in your thoughts... ... deep in your feelings... ... because that is exactly where this land lies, which can become infinitely large in a second...

... ... But in the land of dreams, much more is possible... ... For example, you can determine what the weather should be like... ... maybe a beautiful sunny day that is really nice and warm... ... or you prefer it cool and windy... ... then it can be that way in a second, just like that... ... because you want it that way... ... because you determine it that way... ... So decide for yourself what the weather should be like and observe that it happens exactly like that in the land of your dreams... ... Maybe you know that fantasy and reality are very close together... ... because only what you once thought or imagined as a picture in your fantasy becomes reality...

... ... You approach a crossroads where countless paths converge... ... from all directions, different paths meet here... ... narrow and bumpy... ... wide and comfortable... ... straight and winding... ... leading up and down... ... and also completely level... ... and everywhere there are signs showing where each of these roads leads... ... for each road, for each path, there is a sign shaped like an arrow... ... and on each sign, the destination of the path is written...

... ... You arrive at the crossroads... ... It is huge because infinitely many paths meet here... ... Then you look deeply into the land of dreams and see that the whole land is crisscrossed by these paths... ... But which path should you take

... ... Which one is the right one... ... That is exactly what you may have often asked yourself in your life... ... sometimes finding a quick and good answer... ... sometimes just trusting your feelings... ... Sometimes it was a good path... ... sometimes it was a difficult or arduous... ... or even a very painful path, so you thought it was the wrong path... ... or one you would have preferred to avoid... ... But today you can find the right path... ... the path that leads you to a special goal...

... ... You look at the signs, and they all look the same except for one... ... All signs are bright, only one is dark with black writing... ... You can recognize it immediately because it stands out so clearly from the others... ... You go very close to recognize this different sign... ... It bears the inscription "Death"... ... You know that this is one of the possible paths... ... and that is exactly what you have often thought about recently... ... You know you can take it, and no one could stop you... ... But sometimes it is also the case that people who, like you, think about it are waiting for someone to be there to stop them... ... someone who offers a possibility to continue living and becoming happier again... ... someone who says, "I am here for you"... ... someone you can trust... ... someone who can bear you and accepts you as you are... ... just someone who says, "I am here for you"... ... Maybe you are looking for such a person, or you have already found them and let yourself be carried away by exactly this thought...

... ... To make sure that there are indeed alternatives to death, you now look at the remaining signs, which all look the same... ... You recognize that they all bear the same inscription... ... On each sign at this crossroads, it says "Path to yourself"... ... because all the paths of your life that you walk consciously and with trust can lead to yourself... ... certainly not always easy... ... not always simple or comfortable... ... but always to yourself...

... ... You spontaneously decide on one of the paths that lead to yourself and continue on it... ... You feel deep inside yourself that it is the right path... ... a path into life and thus to yourself...

... ... You go around the next bend, and there are many helpers waiting for you... ... People you know are standing by the roadside, and you might be surprised to see them here as helpers... ... Others you have never seen before... ... but they are there as helpers, and you think about how many people you don't know today can become your companions, help you, and accompany you on a part of your journey... ... So you walk faster and faster... ... as fast as you can, you run across the land of your dreams towards the sun... ... You feel better with every step, and your inner trust in yourself and your helpers grows...

... ... Then you think that your inner helpers are with you every day and that you can meet them deep inside yourself every day... ... ... You think that the land of dreams is deep inside you. It has always been there. I am only telling you about it...

#10

For Affected Individuals

You go into the land of dreams... ... You sit on a comfortable bench, and your gaze sweeps into the distance... ... You can see the land of your dreams and see how vast it is... ... mountains and valleys, rivers and lakes, meadows and forests... ... and deep peace and quiet... ... Maybe you imagined death to be like this or something similar... ... surrounded by peace, completely alone and peaceful... ... That is also how it is here in the land of your dreams - a place where you can find everything you are looking for... ... You think about how, in the past, much of what you wanted to communicate was not understood... ... much of what you wanted to experience was no longer possible... ... some things you would have liked to change were no longer influenceable... ... So you had decided to leave life... ... But you are still here... ... and maybe people have asked you why you did it... ... why you no longer wanted to live...

Maybe many would not understand my words if I tell you that I know you didn't need a reason for it... ... You would have needed one not to do it... ... You would have needed a reason to decide to live... ... Even now, you need this reason, just like all of us... ... You are in the land of dreams to find this reason that makes life worth living... ... even if you may not be able to imagine it well now...

You stand up and wander through the land of your dreams... ... You follow a wide path that leads through this beautiful landscape, past old and gnarled trees... ... up and down hills... ... until you come to a reservoir... ... On the opposite side, a high mountain rises... ... You look at the lake... ... The water is crystal clear, and you can see all the way to the bottom... ... recognizing every stone that lies at the bottom of the lake... ... You find a nice place to rest... ... You sit down, and from your comfortable and quiet spot, you look at the lake... ... The sun reflects silver in it, and the entire surface starts to sparkle... ... You enjoy the peace...

... ... Then slowly pictures rise from the bottom of the lake... ... Pictures of the past slowly float upwards... ... First, a picture of something that once made life worth living rises... ... maybe a success from the past... ... maybe a passion or a special activity... ... a goal or conviction... ... You recognize the picture... ... You see once again what once made life worth living... ... You had lost this feeling, but now you can feel again what it is like when it is worth living... ... You look at the picture in peace and wait until it dissolves on the surface of the lake...

Then more pictures rise... ... Pictures of people you would like to say something to... ... You let their pictures rise and remain completely calm... ... And what you want to say, you shout at the pictures... ... You scream it out of you, as loud as you can... ... You speak it out now... ... Then you wait until the pictures dissolve...

... ... You hear your own voice from the opposite shore like an echo... ... but the voice does not repeat what you shouted... ... It is your own voice calling to you... ... "Start living again!" ...

Then a special picture comes up from the depths... ... one that you cannot directly recognize... ... It shows you what might make it worth living even now... ... The picture comes closer and closer and becomes clearer... ... Maybe you already see it, can already recognize it... ... Perhaps it remains like a mist, but you feel it is here... ... There is this picture, whatever it shows... ... And you still hear your voice like an echo... ... "Start living again!" ...

... ... You dip your hands into the cool water of the lake... ... You let everything that makes it worth living flow through your hands into your body... ... You feel this strength flowing deep into you...

... ... Then you stand up and run across the lake... ... You run so fast that you only now notice that you can walk on water here in the land of your dreams... ... You run to the opposite side and climb the mountain... ... higher and higher... ... until you reach the top of the summit... ... Once at the top, you stand far above everything that could ever hurt and wound you, far above everything that was difficult and hopeless... ... You can see the entire land and shout out everything you have always wanted to say far into the distance... ... You scream it across the land so that everyone can hear you... ... The land belongs to you...

... ... You make yourself comfortable high up on the summit and think about how it was not only your decision to attempt to end your life, it was also your inner decision to survive... ... Somewhere deep inside you, you knew until the last moment and even hoped that someone would find you... ... that someone would pull you out and listen to you... ... take you seriously... ... see you... ... and bear you... ... someone who says, "I am here for you"... ... someone who says, "I will go your way with you"... ... someone who says, "Start living again!" ... ... Today you are here yourself to tell yourself this... ... your own voice calls it to you... ... You yourself give your life the meaning you are looking for... ... You yourself listen to yourself now, as you would have needed from others... ... Your own inner voice whispers to you what you need...

... You resolve to listen to this inner voice every day... ... Then you stand up and roll up your sleeves... ... You have survived, and if you want, you can start living again now... ... Then you think that maybe it is not just like this in the land of dreams, but also in your everyday life... ... Fantasy and reality are much closer together than you thought... ... You think that the land of dreams is deep inside you. It has always been there. I am only telling you about it... ...

Overview of All Titles in the Series "Ten Hypnoses"

Volume 1: Smoking Cessation
Volume 2: Anxiety and Restlessness
Volume 3: Burnout
Volume 4: Reducing Overweight
Volume 5: Coping with the Past
Volume 6: Suicidal Thoughts and Attempts
Volume 7: Psycho-Oncology
Volume 8: Obsessions and Tics
Volume 9: Self-Confidence and Decision-Making
Volume 10: Grief Work
Volume 11: Psychosomatics
Volume 12: Chronic Pain
Volume 13: Depressive Thoughts
Volume 14: Panic Attacks
Volume 15: Domestic Violence, Victim Support
Volume 16: Post-Traumatic Stress
Volume 17: Exam Anxiety and Stage Fright
Volume 18: Anti-Violence Training, Offender Support
Volume 19: Addiction Tendencies
Volume 20: Social Phobia and Fear of Contact
Volume 21: Nail Biting
Volume 22: Self-Awareness and Self-Love
Volume 23: Teeth Grinding and Night Clenching
Volume 24: Feelings of Guilt
Volume 25: Fear in Crowds
Volume 26: Fear of Flying, Aviophobia
Volume 27: Fear in Enclosed Spaces, Claustrophobia
Volume 28: Tinnitus, Ear Noises
Volume 29: Fear of Heights
Volume 30: Neurodermatitis

Volume 31: Finding Inner Balance
Volume 32: Overcoming Loneliness
Volume 33: Fear of Illness, Hypochondria
Volume 34: Anticipatory Anxiety, Fear of Fear
Volume 35: Jealousy in Relationships
Volume 36: Driving Anxiety
Volume 37: New Start after Separation
Volume 38: Fear of Injections
Volume 39: Heart Anxiety Neurosis
Volume 40: Overcoming Resentment and Anger
Volume 41: Resolving Blockages and Positive Thinking
Volume 42: Stress Reduction, Stress Management
Volume 43: Body Relaxation
Volume 44: Deep Relaxation
Volume 45: Fear of the Dark
Volume 46: Falling Asleep and Staying Asleep
Volume 47: Compulsive Buying
Volume 48: Restless Legs Syndrome
Volume 49: Bulimia
Volume 50: Anorexia
Volume 51: Overcoming Nightmares
Volume 52: Imagined Deformity
Volume 53: Overcoming Distrust, Finding Trust
Volume 54: Processing Failures
Volume 55: Humiliation, Emotional Hurt
Volume 56: Distressing Compassion, Vicarious Suffering
Volume 57: Self-Forgiveness
Volume 58: Self-Awareness, Self-Confidence
Volume 59: Saying No
Volume 60: Assertiveness
Volume 61: Setting Boundaries and Self-Assertion
Volume 62: Decision-Making Ability

Volume 63: Success Orientation
Volume 64: Ruminating, Circular Thinking
Volume 65: Accepting Pregnancy
Volume 66: Birth Preparation
Volume 67: Spiritual Opening
Volume 68: Joy of Life and Inner Lightness
Volume 69: Patience and Inner Peace
Volume 70: Fibromyalgia and Rheumatism
Volume 71: Irritable Bowel Syndrome, Crohn's Disease
Volume 72: Fear of Nausea, Emetophobia
Volume 73: Stuttering and Cluttering, Speech Flow Disorders
Volume 74: Concentration and Knowledge Anchoring
Volume 75: Vitality and Spontaneity
Volume 76: Searching for Meaning and Finding Goals
Volume 77: Life Crises, Life Events
Volume 78: Workaholism, Goal Obsession
Volume 79: Helper Syndrome, Helpless Helpers
Volume 80: Medication Abuse
Volume 81: Gambling Addiction
Volume 82: Internet Addiction, Smartphone Addiction
Volume 83: Hoarding Disorder, Compulsive Collecting
Volume 84: Conspiracy Thoughts, Overvalued Ideas
Volume 85: Fear of Operations and Treatments
Volume 86: Fear of Aging
Volume 87: Travel Anxiety
Volume 88: Anxiety When Urinating, Paruresis
Volume 89: Fear of Intimacy and Togetherness
Volume 90: Fear of Blushing
Volume 91: Coming Out in Homosexuality
Volume 92: Charisma Training
Volume 93: Migraines and Chronic Headaches
Volume 94: Overcoming Allergies, Bronchial Asthma

Volume 95: Normalizing Blood Pressure
Volume 96: Compulsive Perfectionism
Volume 97: Sports Hypnosis, Motivation
Volume 98: Sports Hypnosis, Performance Enhancement
Volume 99: Determination and Focus
Volume 100: Encountering the Inner Child
Volume 101: Cravings, Binge Eating
Volume 102: Stimulating Metabolism
Volume 103: Bipolar Mood Swings
Volume 104: Borderline, Identity Crises
Volume 105: Hypomania, Euphoria, Mania
Volume 106: Restlessness, Agitation
Volume 107: Nervous Breakdown
Volume 108: Adjustment Disorders
Volume 109: Self-Alienation, Depersonalization
Volume 110: Ending Self-Pity
Volume 111: Primary Gain of Illness
Volume 112: Secondary Gain of Illness
Volume 113: Bullying, Victim Support
Volume 114: Letting Go of Envy and Jealousy
Volume 115: Fear of Spiders, Arachnophobia
Volume 116: Fear of Dogs or Cats
Volume 117: Fear of Strangers, Xenophobia
Volume 118: Excessive Worries, Generalized Anxiety
Volume 119: Strengthening Sense of Responsibility
Volume 120: Unrequited Love, Heartache
Volume 121: Work-Life Balance
Volume 122: Letting Go of Unattainable Goals
Volume 123: Allowing and Accepting Help
Volume 124: Letting Go of Adult Children
Volume 125: Tourette Syndrome
Volume 126: Life Changes and New Starts

Volume 127: Accepting Life in a Wheelchair
Volume 128: Understanding and Overcoming Homesickness
Volume 129: Understanding and Overcoming Wanderlust
Volume 130: Dizziness, Meniere's Disease
Volume 131: Overcoming Aggression
Volume 132: Cutting and Self-Harm
Volume 133: Hair Pulling, Trichotillomania
Volume 134: Postpartum Depression
Volume 135: For Relatives of Dementia Patients
Volume 136: Self-Harm, Artificial Disorders
Volume 137: Activating Self-Healing Powers
Volume 138: Preventing Depression Relapse
Volume 139: Reactive Psychoses, Follow-Up
Volume 140: Obsessive Thoughts and Impulses
Volume 141: Compulsive Checking
Volume 142: Compulsive Counting, Symmetry Obsession
Volume 143: Compulsive Washing, Cleanliness Obsession
Volume 144: Compulsive Questioning
Volume 145: Dissociative Paralysis
Volume 146: Phantom Pain
Volume 147: Overcoming Complaining
Volume 148: Hay Fever, Pollen Allergy
Volume 149: Sexual Abuse, Victim Support
Volume 150: Standing Strong Against Sexism, #metoo
Volume 151: Binge Eating
Volume 152: Overcoming Thoughts of Revenge
Volume 153: Detachment from the Aggressor, Stockholm Syndrome
Volume 154: Courage to Separate
Volume 155: Chronic Fatigue, Exhaustion
Volume 156: Fear of the Future, Existential Anxiety
Volume 157: Excessive Worry About Children
Volume 158: Fear of Failure

Volume 159: Ending Distrust and Control
Volume 160: Dejection, Dysphoria
Volume 161: Boreout, Chronic Boredom
Volume 162: Bipolar Disorders, Relapse Prevention
Volume 163: Mania, Relapse Prevention
Volume 164: Nihilism, Feelings of Worthlessness
Volume 165: Thumb Sucking
Volume 166: Being Brave
Volume 167: Being Proud
Volume 168: Overcoming Shyness
Volume 169: Being Able to Delegate Responsibility
Volume 170: Being Able to Show Emotions
Volume 171: Letting Go of Guilt, Victim Support
Volume 172: Processing Guilt, Offender Support
Volume 173: Mood Swings, Cyclothymia
Volume 174: Lack of Drive, Vital Sadness
Volume 175: Hearing Voices with Reality Reference
Volume 176: Confident Communication
Volume 177: Standing Up for Oneself
Volume 178: Taking New Paths
Volume 179: Confident Job Application
Volume 180: No Longer Being Taken Advantage Of
Volume 181: End of Submissiveness
Volume 182: Depressive Numbness
Volume 183: Mood Drops, Affective Incontinence
Volume 184: Mood Instability
Volume 185: Somatoform Disorders
Volume 186: Stomach Ulcer, Psychosomatic
Volume 187: Accepting Amputation
Volume 188: Overcoming and Letting Go of Hatred
Volume 189: Ending Accusations
Volume 190: Allowing Tears, Being Able to Cry

Volume 191: Finding and Sorting Repressed Feelings
Volume 192: Somatoform Pain
Volume 193: Living Autonomously
Volume 194: Anhedonia, Joylessness
Volume 195: Persistent Sadness
Volume 196: Obesity, Food Addiction
Volume 197: Parents of Abused Children
Volume 198: Letting Go and Letting Be
Volume 199: Childhood Sexual Abuse
Volume 200: Fear of Loss

www.ingramcontent.com/pod-product-compliance
Lightning Source LLC
Chambersburg PA
CBHW030501220526
45464CB00006B/2609